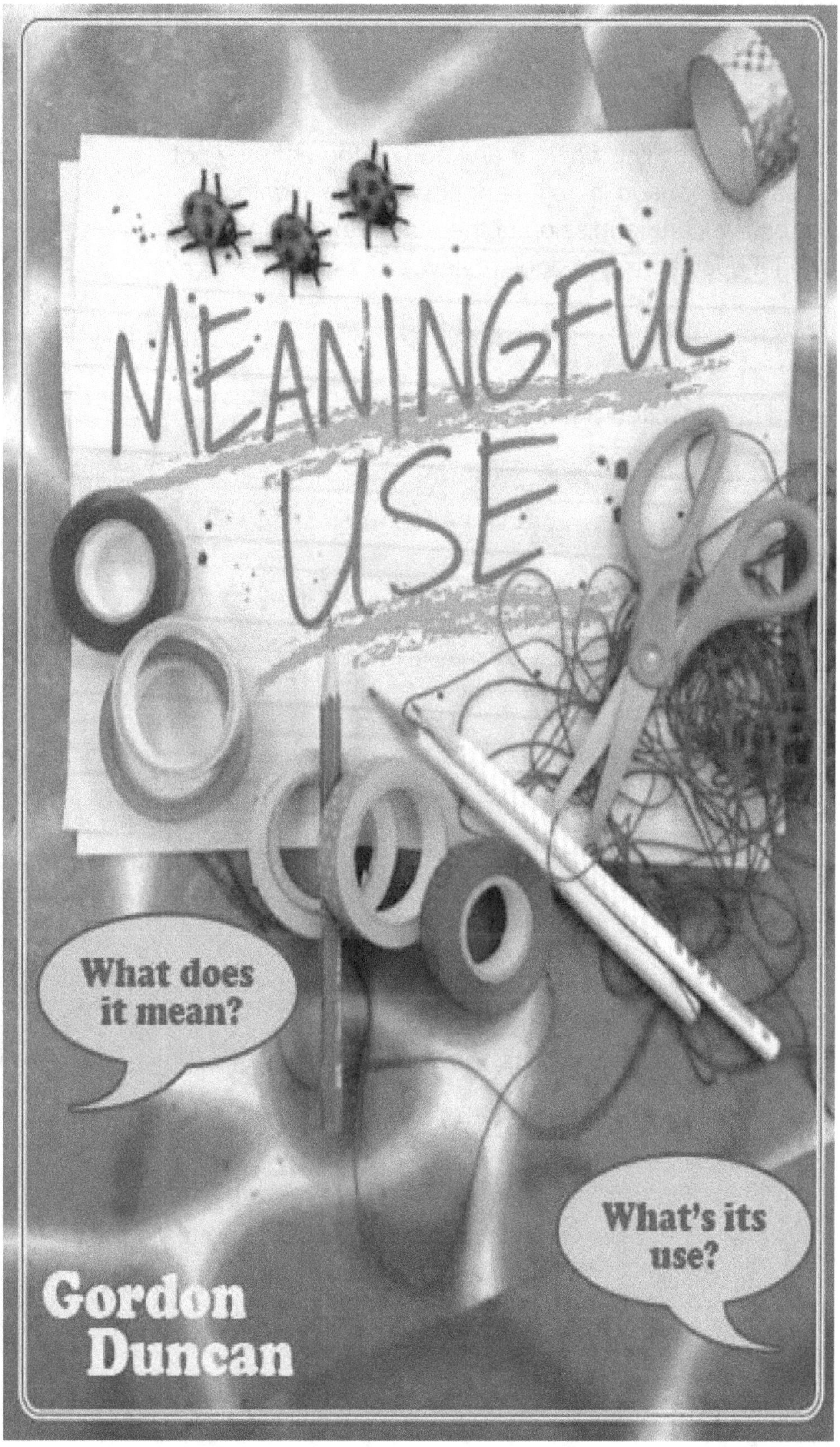

Copyrights

Table of Contents

Preface

There may not be any more confusing (or more pressing) issue for health care providers than understanding and implementing the government's Meaningful Use policies.

In undertaking the research and the writing of this book, I've done my best to find the most accurate and up to date information possible and try to make it simple. I hope you find this relevant and helpful, but I strongly urge each and every possible Eligible Professional to bookmark and return to this site:

http://www.cms.gov/Regulations-and-Guidance/Legislation/EHRIncentivePrograms/

Ultimately, Meaningful Use is intended to enable you to provide more thorough quality care for your patients. That is a goal to get behind and promote. Getting there is the challenge.

So, as you tackle this project, be patient with yourself, recognize that you still have time, and approach it in the way that you do each and every one of your patients: with attention and care.

I hope these pages are helpful.

Gordon Duncan
Practice Progress

What Is Meaningful Use?

What is meaningful use? Well, we live in the era of electronic health records, and while electronic health records can provide many benefits for providers and their patients, those benefits depend on how they're used.

Meaningful use is the set of standards defined by the Centers for Medicare & Medicaid Services (CMS). Included in Meaningful Use are the Incentive Programs that govern the use of electronic health records. They also allow eligible providers and hospitals to earn incentive payments by meeting specific criteria. For details about the incentive programs, visit the CMS website at

http://www.cms.gov/Regulations-and-Guidance/Legislation/EHRIncentivePrograms/index.html?redirect=/EHRIncentivePrograms/.

To bottom line it, the goal of meaningful use is to promote and encourage the spread of electronic health records to improve health care in the United States.

What are the Benefits of Meaningful Use?

There are a host of benefits of the meaningful use of EHRs. They include:

Complete and accurate information

Electronic health records enable providers to have the best information they need to provide the best possible care. Following these guidelines, providers will know even more about their patients that they usually have, and they will have the most up to date health history possible before walking into the examination room.

Better access to information

Electronic health records enable an improved access to the information that providers need to diagnose health problems earlier and to provided healthier outcomes of their patients. Electronic health records also allow that improved information to be shared more easily. Doctors' offices, hospitals, and other health providers will then offer a better coordination of care.

Patient empowerment

Electronic health records will help patients feel empowered to take a greater and more active role in their own health and in the health of their families. Fundamental in this process is the axiom that patients can always receive electronic copies of their medical records, and that will enable them to share that health information over the Internet with their families securely.

How Did We Get Here?

Recently, the government passed the Health Information Technology for Economic and Clinical Health (HITECH) Act.

HITECH provides the Department of Health & Human Services (HHS) with the authority. They have been charged with establishing programs to improve health care quality, safety, and efficiency. They will do this through the promotion of health IT. That health IT will include electronic health records and private and a secure electronic health information exchange between all parties involved.

Under HITECH, health care professionals and hospitals can become eligible to qualify for Medicare and Medicaid incentive payments. They qualify when they adopt certified EHR technology and use it to achieve the specified objectives from HITECH.

So far, there have been four regulations that have been released. Two of them define the "meaningful use" objectives that providers must meet to qualify for the bonus payments, and the other two identify the technical capabilities necessary for EHR technology to be certified.

What are These Incentive Programs?

CMS has issued an Incentive Program for Electronic Health Records. These programs define the minimum requirements that providers must meet through certified EHR technology usage to qualify for the payments for Stages 1, 2 3 of meaningful use.

Incentive Programs

According to cms.gov, "the Medicare and Medicaid EHR Incentive Programs provide incentive payments to eligible professionals, eligible hospitals and critical access hospitals (CAHs) as they adopt, implement, upgrade or demonstrate meaningful use of certified EHR technology."

How much can be earned?

According to cms.gov, EP's can receive up to $44,000 through the Medicare EHR Incentive Program and up to $63,750 through the Medicaid EHR Incentive Program.

Qualifier

According to cms.gov, incentive payments made through the Medicare Electronic Health Records (EHR) Incentive Program are subject to the mandatory reductions in federal spending known as sequestration, required by the Budget Control Act of 2011.

The American Taxpayer Relief Act of 2012 postponed sequestration for 2 months. As required by law, President Obama issued a sequestration order on March 1, 2013. Under these mandatory reductions, Medicare EHR incentive payments made to eligible professionals and eligible hospitals will be reduced by 2%. This 2% reduction will be applied to any Medicare EHR incentive payment for a reporting period that ends on or after April 1, 2013. If the final day of the reporting period occurs before April 1, 2013, those incentive payments will not be subject to the reduction.

Please note that this reduction does not apply to Medicaid EHR incentive payments, which are exempt from the mandatory reductions.

Medicare Incentive Program

The Medicare EHR Incentive Program provides incentive payments to EP's, eligible hospitals, and CAHs that are capable and able to demonstrate meaningful use of certified EHR technology.

EP's can receive up to $44,000 over five years under the Medicare EHR Incentive Program.

There's an additional incentive for EP's who provide services in a Health Professional Shortage Area (HSPA).To get the maximum incentive payment, Medicare eligible professionals must begin participation by 2012.

Who are the Eligible Professionals in the Medicare Incentive Program?

According to cms.gov, these are the practitioners who may participate in the Medicare program.

Doctor of medicine or osteopathy

Doctor of dental surgery or dental medicine

Doctor of podiatry

Doctor of optometry

Chiropractor

Medicaid Incentive Program

The Medicaid EHR Incentive Program provides incentive payments to EP's, eligible hospitals, and CAHs as they adopt, implement, upgrade, or demonstrate meaningful use of certified EHR technology in their first year of participation. They are then required to demonstrate meaningful use for the five remaining participation years.

EP's can receive up to $63,750 over the six years that they choose to participate in the program

The Medicaid EHR Incentive Program is voluntarily offered by 43 individual states and territories, and more states will begin offering the program in 2012.

If you do not know whether your state is participating, check with your State Medicaid Agency for more information.

Who are the Eligible Professionals in the Medicaid Incentive Program?

According to cms.gov, these are the practitioners who may participate in the Medicaid program.

Physicians (primarily doctors of medicine and doctors of osteopathy)

Nurse practitioner

Certified nurse-midwife

Dentist

Physician assistant who furnishes services in a Federally Qualified Health Center of Rural Health Clinic that is led by a physician assistant.

What is EHR?

An electronic health record (EHR)—sometimes called an electronic medical record (EMR) enables healthcare providers to record patient information electronically instead of being completely dependent on using paper records.

But EHRs are often capable of doing much more than just recording information. Participation in the EHR Incentive Program asks providers to use the capabilities of their EHRs to achieve government determined benchmarks that are intended to lead to improved patient care.

An important disclaimer to understand is that the EHR Incentive Program is NOT a reimbursement program for purchasing or replacing an EHR.

Providers have to meet specific requirements in order to receive incentive payments.

Stages of Meaningful Use

Stage 1 Data capture and sharing

Stage 1 covered the years 2011-2012. Stage 1 Meaningful Use criteria focused on several things. They are/were:

Electronically capturing health information in a standardized format.

Using that information to track key clinical conditions.

Communicating that information for care coordination processes.

Initiating the reporting of clinical quality measures and public health information.

Using information to engage patients and their families in their care.

Stage 2 Advance clinical processes

Stage 2 will be initiated in 2014. Stage 2 Meaningful Use criteria also focuses on several things. They are:

More rigorous health information exchange (HIE).

Increased requirements for e-prescribing and incorporating lab results.

Electronic transmission of patient care summaries across multiple settings.

More patient-controlled data.

Stage 3 Improved outcomes

Stage 3 will be initiated in 2016. Stage 3 Meaningful Use criteria also focuses on several things. They are:

Improving quality, safety, and efficiency, leading to improved health outcomes.

Decision support for national high-priority conditions.

Patient access to self-management tools.

Access to comprehensive patient data through patient-centered HIE.

Improving population health.

How Eligible Professionals (EP) Achieve Meaningful Use (MU)?

In order to achieve MU, an EP will need to do three things.

They will need to use certified Electronic Health Record (EHR) technology.

They will need to use technology for the electronic exchange of health information to improve their quality of care.

They will need to report on Clinical Quality Measures (CQMs).

Questions Surrounding Eligibility

The above criteria may raise more questions than answers so let's try to answer some of those questions.

Are hospital based professionals eligible for incentives?

No, they are not.

How is a hospital defined?

Hospitals are those in which covered services in an inpatient (POS 21) or emergency room (POS 23) equal 90% or more.

Are incentives based on individual or practice performance?

Incentives are based on individual performance, not practice performance.

Can a provider be eligible through both Medicare and Medicaid?

A provider can be eligible for incentives only through one or the other. They can only participate in one program.

What are the eligibility criteria for Medicaid?

An EP must have more than 30% of their patient volume covered by Medicaid.

A pediatrician only needs more than 20%.

The practice must predominantly be in a federal or rural health center.

They EP must be licensed and credentialed with no OIG exclusions.

What are the eligibility criteria for Medicare?

An EP must have Part B Medicare allowed charges.

An EP must be enrolled in PECOS system (CMS provider enrollment system), living.

What is required in Stage 1?
First: 15 Core Objectives

All 15 core objectives are required. What are they, and how will they be measured?

Core Objective One:

EPs must enable users to electronically record, modify, and retrieve patient demographic data including preferred language, gender, race, ethnicity, and date of birth.

How will it be measured?

More than 50% of all an EP's unique patients must have their demographics recorded as structured data.

Core Objective Two:

EP's must maintain their patients' active medication list

How will it be measured?

An EP must have more than 80% of all their unique patients documented with at least one entry recorded as structured data (or there must be an indication that the patient is not currently prescribed any medication).

Core Objective Three:

EP's must maintain their patient's active medication allergy list.

How will it be measured?

An EP must have more than 80% of all their unique patients documented with at least one entry recorded as structured data (or there must be an indication that the patient has no known medication allergies).

Core Objective Four:

An EP must record and chart changes in the following vital signs:

Height

Weight

Blood pressure

Calculate and display: BMI

Plot and display growth charts for children 2–20 years, including BMI.

How will it be measured?

An EP must have more than 50% of all unique patients from age 2 and over recorded with height, weight, and blood pressure as structured data.

Core Objective Five:

An EP must record smoking status for patients 13 years old or older.

How will it be measured?

An EP must have documented the smoking status of more than 50% of all unique patients 13 years old or older as structured data.

Core Objective Six:

An EP must keep and maintain an up-to-date problem list of current and active diagnoses based on ICD–9–CM or SNOMED CT®.

How will it be measured?

An EP must have documented more than 80% of all unique patients with at least one entry or there must be an indication that there are no known problems for the patient recorded as structured data

Core Objective Seven:

An EP must keep a Computerized physician order entry (CPOE) of medications

How will it be measured?

An EP must have documented more than 30% of their unique patients with at least one medication in their medication list with at least one medication order entered using CPOE.

Core Objective Eight:

An EP must conduct Drug-drug and drug-allergy interaction checks.

How will it be measured?

An EP must have enabled this functionality for the entire EHR reporting period.

Core Objective Nine:

An EP must generate and transmit permissible prescriptions electronically (eRx).

How will it be measured?

An EP must transmit more than 40% of all permissible prescriptions written electronically.

Core Objective Ten:

An EP must implement at least one clinical decision support rule.

How will it be measured?

An EP must implement at least one clinical decision support rule relevant to specialty or high clinical priority. That EP must also possess the ability to track and demonstrate compliance for that rule.

Core Objective Eleven:

An EP must possess the capability to exchange key clinical information among other providers of care and with other patient-authorized entities electronically.

How will it be measured?

An EP must have performed at least one successful test to electronically exchange key clinical information.

Core Objective Twelve:

An EP must provide clinical summaries for their patients for each office visit.

How will it be measured?

An EP must provide clinical summaries for more than 50% of patients for all office visits within three business days.

Core Objective Thirteen:

Upon request, an EP must provide patients with an electronic copy of their health information.

How will it be measured?

An EP must provide health information in an electronic copy for more than 50% of all patients who request it. It must be provided within three business days of the request.

Core Objective Fourteen:

An EP must report a total of 6 ambulatory clinical quality measures to CMS (Medicare EHR Incentive Program) or States (Medicaid EHR Incentive Program).

How will it be measured?

For 2011, an EP must provide aggregate numerator, denominator, and exclusions through attestation as discussed in section II(A)(3) of this final rule.

For 2012, an EP must electronically submit the clinical quality measures as discussed in section II(A)(3) of this final rule.

Core Objective Fifteen:

An EP must protect electronic health information created or maintained by the certified EHR technology through the implementation of appropriate technical capabilities.

How will it be measured?

An EP must conduct or review a security risk analysis per 45 CFR 164.308 (a)(1). If necessary, an EP must implement security updates and correct identified security deficiencies as part of their risk management process.

What is required in Stage 1?
Second: 5 of 10 menu objectives are required.

Eligible Professionals must meet 5 of the following 10 core objectives.

Menu Objective One:

Drug-formulary checks

How will it be measured?

An EP has enabled functionality of drug-formulary checks. The EP also has access to at least one internal or external formulary for the entire EHR reporting period.

Menu Objective Two:

Incorporate clinical lab test results as structured data

How will it be measured?

An EP will have incorporated more than 40 percent of all clinical lab test results ordered during the EHR reporting period whose results are either in a positive/negative or numerical format in certified EHR technology as structured data.

Menu Objective Three:

Generate lists of patients by specific conditions

How will it be measured?

An EP must generate at least one report listing patients with a specific condition.

Menu Objective Four:

Send reminders to patients per patient preference for preventive/follow up care

How will it be measured?

An EP will have sent more than 20 percent of all patients 65 years or older or 5 years old or younger an appropriate reminder during the EHR reporting period.

Menu Objective Five:

Provide patients with timely electronic access to their health information

How will it be measured?

An EP must provide timely (available to the patient within four business days of being updated in the certified EHR technology) electronic access to the health information of at least 10 percent of all unique patients. The request is subject to the EP's discretion to withhold certain information.

Menu Objective Six:

Use certified EHR technology to identify patient-specific education resources and provide to patient, if appropriate

How will it be measured?

An EP must provide patient-specific educational resources to more than 10 percent of all unique patients.

Menu Objective Seven:

Medication reconciliation

How will it be measured?

An EP must perform medication reconciliation for more than 50 percent of transitions of care when a patient is transitioned into the care of an EP.

Menu Objective Eight:

Summary of care record for each transition of care/referrals

How will it be measured?

An EP must provide a summary of care record for more than 50 percent of transitions of care and referrals when that EP transitions or refers their patients to another setting of care or provider.

Menu Objective Nine:

Capability to submit electronic data to immunization registries/systems*

How will it be measured?

An EP must have performed at least one test of certified EHR technology's capacity to submit electronic data to immunization registries. They must also follow up that submission if the test is successful (unless none of the immunization registries to which the EP submits such information has the capacity to receive the information electronically).

Menu Objective Ten:

Capability to provide electronic syndromic surveillance data to public health agencies*

How will it be measured?

An EP must have performed at least one test of certified EHR technology's capacity to provide electronic syndromic surveillance data to public health agencies and follow-up submission if the test is successful (unless none of the public health agencies to which an EP submits information has the capacity to receive the information electronically).

* At least 1 public health objective must be selected

What is required in Stage 1?
Third : Clinical Quality Measures

What are the Meaningful Use Stage 1 Clinical Quality Measures?

The objective set forth in the Meaningful Use Stage 1 final rule is that EP's and hospitals must be able to record, store, and report clinical quality measures (CQM).

CMS defines CQM as the "processes, experience, and/or outcomes of patient care, observations or treatment that relate to one or more quality aims for health care such as effective, safe, efficient, patient-centered, equitable, and timely care."

If that is not entirely clear, cms.gov defines them as in this way:

Quality measures are tools that help us measure or quantify healthcare processes, outcomes, patient perceptions, and organizational structure and/or systems that are associated with the ability to provide high-quality health care and/or that relate to one or more quality goals for health care. These goals include: effective, safe, efficient, patient-centered, equitable, and timely care.

How are they collected and reported?

According to cms.gov, data on quality measures are collected or reported in a variety of ways, such as claims, assessment instruments, chart abstraction, registries.

CMS is currently testing the submission of quality measures data from Electronic Health Records for physicians and other health care professionals and will soon be testing with hospitals.

What makes one eligible?

Eligible professionals must report from the table of 44 clinical quality measures which includes, 3 Core, 3 Alternate Core, and 38 additional CQM.

EP's must report on the 3 required core CQMs, and if the denominator of 1 or more of the required core measures is 0, then eligible professionals are permitted to report results for up to 3 alternate core measures.

EP's must also select 3 additional CQMs from a set of 38 CQMs (excluding the core/alternate core measures). For these additional measures, it is acceptable to have a '0' denominator provided the EP does not have an applicable population.

What are the 3 Core Measures?

Adult Weight Screening and Follow up

Preventive Care and Screening Measure Pair:

> Tobacco Use Assessment
> Tobacco Cessation Intervention

Hypertension: Blood Pressure Measurement

What are the 3 Alternative Core Measures?

Weight Assessment and Counseling for Children and Adolescents

Preventive Care and Screening: Influenza Immunization for Patients 50 Years Old or Older

Childhood Immunization Status

What are the 38 Additional Measures?

Diabetes: Hemoglobin A1c Poor Control

Diabetes: Low Density Lipoprotein (LDL) Management and control

Diabetes: Blood Pressure Management

Heart Failure (HF): Angiotensin-Converting Enzyme (ACE) Inhibitor or Angiotensin Receptor Blocker (ARB) Therapy for Left Ventricular Systolic Dysfunction (LSVD)

Coronary Artery Disease (CAD): Beta-Blocker Therapy for CAD Patients with Prior Myocardial Infarction

Pneumonia Vaccination Status for Older Adults

Breast Cancer Screening Description

Colorectal Cancer Screening Description

Coronary Artery Disease (CAD): Oral Antiplatelet Therapy Prescribed for Patients with CAD

Heart Failure (HF): Beta-Blocker Therapy for Left Ventricular Systolic Dysfunction (LVSD)

Anti-depressant medication management:

    Effective Acute Phase Treatment
    Effective Continuation Phase Treatment

Primary Open Angle Glaucoma (POAG): Optic Nerve Evaluation

Diabetic Retinopathy: Documentation of Presence or Absence of Macular Edema and Level of Severity of Retinopathy

Diabetic Retinopathy: Communication with the Physician Managing Ongoing Diabetes Care

Asthma Pharmacologic Therapy

Asthma Assessment

Appropriate Testing for Children with Pharyngitis

Oncology Breast Cancer: Hormonal Therapy for Stage IC-IIIC Estrogen Receptor/Progesterone Receptor (ER/PR) Positive Breast Cancer

Oncology Colon Cancer: Chemotherapy for Stage III Colon Cancer Patients

Prostate Cancer: Avoidance of Overuse of Bone Scan for Staging Low Risk Prostate Cancer Patients

Smoking and Tobacco Use Cessation, Medical assistance:

> Advising Smokers and Tobacco Users to Quit
> Discussing Smoking and Tobacco Use Cessation Medications
> Discussing Smoking and Tobacco Use Cessation Strategies

Diabetes: Eye Exam

Diabetes: Urine Screening

Diabetes: Foot Exam

Coronary Artery Disease (CAD): Drug Therapy for Lowering LDL Cholesterol

Heart Failure (HF): Warfarin Therapy Patients with Atrial Fibrillation

Ischemic Vascular Disease (IVD): Blood Pressure Management

Ischemic Vascular Disease (IVD): Use of Aspirin or Another Antithrombotic

Initiation and Engagement of Alcohol and Other Drug Dependence Treatment:

    Initiation
    Engagement

Prenatal Care: Screening for Human Immunodeficiency Virus (HIV)

Prenatal Care: Anti-D Immune Globulin

Controlling High Blood Pressure

Cervical Cancer Screening

Chlamydia Screening for Women

Use of Appropriate Medications for Asthma

Ischemic Vascular Disease (IVD): Complete Lipid Panel and LDL Control

Diabetes: Hemoglobin A1c Control (<8.0%)

Low Back Pain: Use of Imaging Studies

Important Dates

In the midst of all of this confusion, perhaps the most important question is, "When and how do I need to implement all of this?"

Here are some important dates that apply to receiving the maximum incentive possible.

January 1, 2013

This is the date that EP's must begin their reporting year.

October 3, 2013

This is the last day that EP's can begin the 90-day reporting period for calendar year 2013 for the Medicare EHR Incentive Program.

Note: If EP's attested in 2011 or 2012, this is not applicable.

December 31, 2013

This is the end of the EP reporting year.

February 28, 2014

This is the last day for eligible EP's to register and attest to receive an incentive payment for calendar year 2013.

2015

Medicare payment adjustments begin for EP's that are not meaningful users of HER technology.

2016

This is the last year to receive a Medicare EHR Incentive payment.

This is the also the last year to initiate participation in the Medicaid EHR Incentive Program.

2021

This is the last year to receive a Medicaid EHR Incentive payment.

How are the Medicare and Medicaid Programs Different?

Implementation

Medicare

The Federal Government will implement this program as an option nationally.

Medicaid

This will be voluntary for states to implement (but some states may not have any choice).

Payment Reductions

Medicare

Payment reductions begin in 2015 for providers that do not demonstrate Meaningful Use.

Medicaid

There will be no Medicaid payment reductions.

Demonstration

Medicare

You much demonstrate Meaningful Use in Year One.

Medicaid

Each state can adopt their own certain additional requirements for Meaningful Use.

Initiation Deadline

Medicare

The last year a provider may initiate the program is 2014.

Medicaid

The last year a provider may initiate the program is 2016.

Registration Deadline

Medicare

The last year to register is 2016. Payment adjustments begin in 2015.

Medicaid

The last year to register is 2016.

Where Can I Find More Help?

CMS Official Website

You can find detailed information, tip sheets and more at CMS' official website for the EHR incentive programs:

http://www.cms.gov/EHRIncentivePrograms

EHR Incentive Twitter Feed

You can follow the latest information about the HER Incentive Programs on Twitter at:

http://www.Twitter.com/CMSGov

Certification Support

You can learn more about certification and certified EHRs, in addition to other ONC programs that are designed to give support to providers during the transition at:

http://healthit.hhs.gov

CMS Tipsheet

To find helpful tips to guide you along the way, visit:

http://www.cms.gov/Regulations-and-Guidance/Legislation/EHRIncentivePrograms/Downloads/ClinicalQualityMeasuresTipsheet.pdf

Acronym Guide for the EHR Program

ACA - Patient Protection and Affordable Care Act

A/I/U - Adopt, implement, or upgrade

CAH - Critical Access Hospital

CCN - CMS Certification Number

CHIPRA – Children's Health Insurance Program Reauthorization Act of 2009

CMS - Centers for Medicare & Medicaid Services

CNM - Certified Nurse Midwife

CPOE - Computerized Physician Order Entry

CQM – Clinical Quality Measures

CY – Calendar Year

HER - Electronic Health Record

EP – Eligible Professional

eRx – E-Prescribing

FFS – Fee – for -service

FQHC – Federally Qualified Health Center

FFY – Federal Fiscal Year

HHS – U.S. Department of Health and Human Services

HIT – Health Information Technology

HITECH Act – Health Information Technology for Economic and Clinical Health Act

HITPC – Health Information Technology Policy Committee

HIPAA – Health Insurance Portability and Accountability Act of 1996

HPSA – Health Professional Shortage Area

MA – Medicare Advantage

MCMP – Medicare Care Management Performance Demonstration

MU – Meaningful Use

NCVHS – National Committee on Vital and Health Statistics

NP – Nurse Practitioner

NPI – National Provider Identifier

NPRM – Notice of Proposed Rulemaking

OMB – Office of Management and Budget

ONC – Office of the National Coordinator of Health Information Technology

PA – Physician Assistant

PECOS – Provider Enrollment, Chain, and Ownership System

PPS – Prospective Payment System (Part A)

PQRI – Medicare Physician Quality Reporting Initiative

Recovery Act – American Reinvestment & Recovery Act of 2009

RHC – Rural Health Clinic

RHQDAPU – Reporting Hospital Quality Data for Annual Payment Update

TIN – Taxpayer Identification Number

About the Author

Gordon Duncan is an award-winning educator, salesman, teacher, manager, and writer. He has taught in the public school system, lobbied for school's accreditation, managed eye clinics, led sales' teams, and also publishes books on theology, church, and culture.

You can find out more about his philosophies for the eye industry at www.practiceprogress.com and his thoughts on church and culture at www.jgordonduncan.com.

www.ingramcontent.com/pod-product-compliance
Lightning Source LLC
Chambersburg PA
CBHW081403170526
45166CB00010B/3186